Nature's Universal Healer.

Formulae & Recipes.

By

Dr. Patricia W. Alex

Copyright 2021. All rights reserved

Table of Contents.

- CHAPTER ONE. 6
- INTRODUCTION TO DMSO (DIMETHYLSULFOXIDE).........6
- CHAPTER TWO. 9
- WHAT IS DMSO (DIMETHYLSULFOXIDE)? 9
- CHAPTER THREE. 11
- HISTORY AND CONTROVERSY OF DMSO......................11
  - What Went Wrong? 12
- CHAPTER FOUR. 15
- CHEMICAL COMPOSITION OF DMSO. 15
  - METHODS OF APPLYING DMSO. 16
    - Topical (on the skin) Method: 16
    - Oral (through the mouth) Method. 17
    - Intravenous (injection) Method. 18
- CHAPTER FIVE. 20
- CLINICAL BENEFITS OF DMSO. 20
  - TOXIC EFFECT OF DMSO. 22
- CHAPTER SIX. 28
- USING DMSO THERAPHY FOR TREATING AILMENTS. 28
    - DMSO THERAPY FOR AMYLIODOSIS. 28
  - *Dosage Application;* 31
    - DMSO THERAPY FOR TREATING ARTHRITIS........32

Dosage Application; 34

- DMSO THERAPY FOR TREATING ACHES AND NERVE PAIN. 34

Dosage Application; 36

- DMSO FOR SPORT INJURIES. 37

Dosage Application; 39

- DMSO FOR BRAIN INJURIES. 39
- DMSO THERAPY FOR TREATING BURNS. 43
- DMSO THERAPY FOR TREATING CANCER. 45

Dosage Application; 46

- DMSO THERAPY FOR DIABETES. 47

Dosage Application; 48

- DMSO THERAPY FOR DIGESTIVE PROBLEMS. 48
- DMSO THERAPY FOR EYE AILMENTS. 51

Dosage Application. 54

- DMSO THERAPY FOR TREATING EAR AND HEARING PROBLEMS. 54

Dosage Application. 56

- DMSO THERAPY FOR FUNGUS INFECTIONS. 56

Dosage Application. 57

- DMSO THERAPY FOR HAIR GROWTH AND SCALP PROBLEMS. 58

Dosage Application; 60

- DMSO THERAPY HEADACHES AND MIGRAINES. .60

Dosage Application; 62

- DMSO THERAPY FOR INFLAMMATION. 63

Dosage Application; 64

- DMSO THERAPY FOR MENTAL ILLNESS AND RETARDATION. 65

Dosage Application; 66

- DMSO THERAPY FOR SKIN AILMENT. 66

Dosage Application; 67

- DMSO THERAPY FOR SHINGLES AND HERPES. ...68

Dosage Application; 70

- DMSO FOR STROKE, SPINAL CORD INJURIES. 70

Dosage Application; 72

CHAPTER SEVEN. 73

POSSIBLE SIDE EFFECTS OF DMSO. 73

DMSO MIXTURE QUANTITY & DOSAGE. 74

- For 50/50 percent solution: 74
- 70/30 percent solution: 74
- 10/90 percent solution: 75

CHAPTER EIGHT. 76

PRECAUTIONARY MEASURES OF DMSO FOR
PREGNANT WOMEN AND NURSING MOTHERS. 76

- REASONS FOR STORING AND MIXING DMSO. 77

OTHER PRECAUTIONARY MEASURES IN THE USE OF
DMSO. 79

- Skin Irritation. 79
- Clean the Skin. 80
- Taste of DMSO. 81
- Dangers For Children. 81
- Dosage Measures. 82
- DMSO With Alcohol. 82
- DMSO And It's Odour. 83

CHAPTER NINE. 84
CONCLUSION. 84

CHAPTER ONE.

INTRODUCTION TO DMSO (DIMETHYLSULFOXIDE)

Dimethyl sulfoxide is a colorless liquid obtained as a by-product of wood pulp when making paper. This colorless liquid has been found to be rapidly used as a dipolar aprotic solvent miscible (capable of being mixed) with water with the capability of eliminating huge catalog of small and foreign molecules.

DMSO is a multi-versatile healing therapy that tends to cure virtually all ailments ever known. DMSO is used oftentimes to reduce pain and speed up the treatment of wounds, burns, muscle and bone injuries. DMSO is also used topically to treat painful conditions such as headaches, inflammation, osteoarthritis, rheumatoid arthritis, and severe facial pain called tic douloureux (a severe pain on one side of the face).

It is used for treating certain eye conditions such as, glaucoma, cataracts and retina problems; for foot ailments like bunions (a bony bump that forms on the joint at the base of your big toe), callus (a thickened layers on the skin; either on the hand or feet), and fungus on the toes; and for skin conditions like keloid scars (a raised scar after an injury has healed maybe be as a result of excess protein in the skin during the healing process) and scleroderma (hard skin). It is sometimes used to treat skin and tissue damage caused by chemotherapy.

DMSO can be used alone or in combination with idoxuridine (an antiviral drug) to treat pains associated with shingles (herpes zoster infection – a reactivation of chickenpox virus in the body).

By injection, DMSO is used to lower abnormally high blood pressure in the brain. It is also prescribed for the treatment of bladder infections (internal cystitis) and chronic inflammatory bowel disease. The Food & Drug

Administration (FDA) in the United States of America, has approved certain DMSO implants to treat symptoms of chronic inflammation. DMSO is sometimes injected into bile ducts and other drugs to treat bile duct stones and several others. Given its useful properties as an anti-inflammatory agent and an active anti-inflammatory agent, dimethyl sulfoxide has the potential to be used in a very wide dose.

This topical agent (DMSO) has long been recognized for treatments beyond the skin. In addition to the diagnostic benefits offered, in many cases, treatment can be applied directly to disease outbreaks.

This book discusses the history, chemical and clinical use of this single agent — dimethyl sulfoxide (DMSO) — and a common controversial past. It is widely used as a keratolytic agent (for removing thick scale on the skin) in combination with potassium hydroxide (KOH) to improve the detection of fungal hyphae.

CHAPTER TWO.

WHAT IS DMSO (DIMETHYLSULFOXIDE)?

The Dimethyl sulfoxide (DMSO) is a drug prescribed by medical professionals such as doctors that can be used as a dietary supplement which are taken either orally (by the mouth), applied directly to the skin (topically) or intravenously using injections or drip. It is often used in the treatment of several ailments such as amylodosis (diseases that result from abnormal insertion of proteins into the organs or tissues). It is basically a smelly solvent with variety of medical uses.

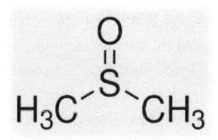

Dimethyl sulfoxide (DMSO) is popularly known as a "miracle" drug with many medicinal properties with diverse biological actions. It has several amazing properties that can be useful in treating many medical ailments. DMSO is a naturally occurring compound. In 1963, a study showed that this paper-making by-product had some amazing properties, including rapid penetration of the skin, distribution of other drugs to the biological tissue, local anesthetics, reducing inflammation and promoting treatment. The first release of the Investigational New Drug (IND) about DMSO study in humans was brought to light by the Food and Drug Administration in 1963. However, lack of controlled studies and the extensive use of DMSO till 1965 led to many unconventional treatments including DMSO. In November 1965 the FDA discontinued all DMSO clinical studies because toxic studies showed that DMSO causes discoloration in the eye experimented animals.

CHAPTER THREE.

HISTORY AND CONTROVERSY OF DMSO.

Like many modern medical products, DMSO derives its roots from the newly developed German chemical industry in the late 19th century. In search of cheaper, more efficient ways of making paper out of wood chips, a process was developed in which its derivatives incorporated different types of sulfides.

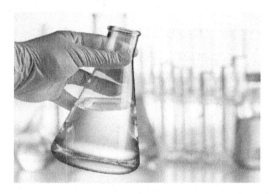

The history of DMSO as a pharmaceutical agent began in 1961 while exploring its potency as an anesthetic, it was discovered that it passed through the skin quickly and deeply without damaging it. Its capacity to pass through the skin is not only because it is a very cool molecule, but also because it has two methyl groups that relate strongly with fats in the skin. Another danger associated with DMSO is that although it may not be considered toxic itself, it is very effective in transmitting other toxic substances into the body through skin contact. These harmful sulfides are converted to less harmful sulfoxides, including DMSO.

Haven gained its approval from the U.S Food and Drug Administration (FDA) 2016 after its discovery in 1961, DMSO became widely known by reporters, pharmaceutical industries and patients with various medical complain.

What Went Wrong?

However, since DMSO was generally obtainable as a solvent and a chemical compound (instead of a banned drug), patients no longer seek for doctor's prescription for it. Therefore, many patients began taking it on their own, often unaware of the right dose or side effects.

Due to this uncontrolled treatment, the FDA has not been able to ensure that its experiments and use are safe. The medical community became disappointed, and this singular act led to the bad reputation given to DMSO all the while.

This controversy was further escalated when it was reported that a woman of Irish origin died of allergies after consuming DMSO with other drugs. Although the exact cause of her death wasn't known, but media reported DMSO as the cause.

About the same time laboratory animals that were given DMSO doses much higher than those that would be given to humans generated deformities in their lenses. After Two months all clinical trials of DMSO in the United States was later shut down by the FDA, using the death of the Irish woman and the negative findings from animal tests as their basis of conclusion.

But in the last 20 years, with hundreds of laboratory and human studies, no more deaths and changes in human eyes have been recorded. In 2016 the EPA finally approved DMSO for medical use in the US, ultimately opening up more potential uses. DMSO is widely used as a local painkiller, as an anti-inflammatory, and antioxidant. It is often mixed with antibiotics, which enable them to penetrate the skin as well as the toe and finger nails.

CHAPTER FOUR.

CHEMICAL COMPOSITION OF DMSO.

Dimethyl sulfoxide is a Dipolar organic compound, *weighing 78.13* is a stable, colorless, immature, hydroscopic liquid, highly sensitive to sulfur-like odors and with a slightly bitter taste.

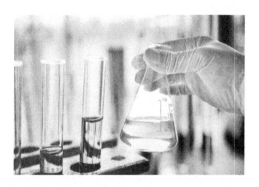

DMSO is completely incomprehensible to water by any measure and acts as a hydrogen bond. DMSO can interact with a wide range of chemicals including: metal cat-ions, different drugs, and tissue components, blood, plasma, spinal fluid etc.

DMSO can act as an oxidizing and as well as a reducing agent. As an oxidant, DMSO is reduced to dimethyl sulfide (DMS) and as a reducing agent, DMSO is attached to dimethyl sulfone (DMSO).

METHODS OF APPLYING DMSO.

There are generally 3 methods of applying DMSO. These include:

- **Topical (on the skin) Method:**

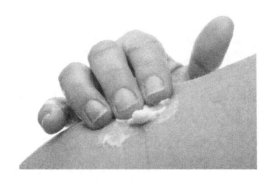

Using this method of application, DMSO helps reduce the incidence of pain, as well as enable recovery from burns, cuts and muscle injuries. It is also used topically to other treatment ailments such as headaches, inflammation, diabetes, eye problems and several others that will be discussed in this book.

DMSO is usually administered in a gel or liquid form on the skin surface. The liquid tends to be more effective although some persons prefer using the gel to the liquid.

- **<u>Oral (through the mouth) Method.</u>**

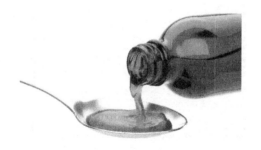

The traditional oral dosage use of DMSO is one to two teaspoons a day. Considering the strong and foul taste of DMSO, it is mixed with tomato juice, grape juice, or any other tasty beverage that can help subsidize its foul taste.

DMSO has this garlic-like taste in the mouth when taken and there's of having this smell in your skin.

- **<u>Intravenous (injection) Method.</u>**

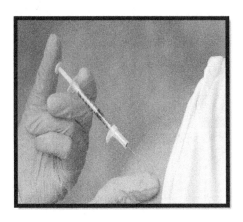

When administered intravenously, DMSO is used to reduce abnormally high blood pressure in the brain. It can also be used to treat interstitial cystitis (infection of the bladder) as well as chronic inflammation of the bladder.

DMSO is often times administered inside the bile duct along with other medications to treat bile duct stones and other ailments.

CHAPTER FIVE.

CLINICAL BENEFITS OF DMSO.

Amid the various sulfur compounds, one can say that DMSO is the only sulfur compound with a wide variety of healing therapeutical value. Contrary to chemical elements capable of restricting the presentation of symptoms, rather than recover those symptoms or weaken the body, DMSO is of the natural remedies which help to promote and strengthen the healing systems embedded in the body.

The best technique to all medicines; either ***natural or artificial,*** is applying the right dosage and appropriate usage.

It is generally known that certain substances, or regularly used drugs seen everywhere such as ibuprofen or acetaminophen, can be misused or overused by people. Depending on different individual's health status, different people may show several reactions or no response at all when same dosage of same drug is used.

Its main use is to convey other drugs across the skin, including drugs such as morphine sulfate, penicillin, steroids and cortisone. It can also serve as a local aneasthetic, which help reduce pains by obstructing outer nerve fibers. Burns, cuts, and bruises are also treated using DMSO, and the relief is almost instantly because it is an antioxidant. DMSO can also be used to reduce inflammation. Examples, it relieves people with symptoms of rheumatoid arthritis and chronic inflammatory bowel disease, toxic immune syndromes, or any other form of self-harm.

DMSO can also be used as a quivering agent to help patients with stroke, and also reduce intracranial pressure in patients with severe head disturbance. It can be used to treat soft tissue injuries, local tissue loss, skin ulcers, and also serve as a delaying factor to the spread of certain types of cancer.

Excitingly, due to the antioxidant properties embedded in DMSO, can be used to reduce some of the effects of aging as well. Furthermore, DMSO is effective for;

- Inflammation bladder disease
- Pains caused by shingels
- Bile duct stones.
- Cancer-related pain
- Foot ulcers associated with diabetes.
- High blood pressure in the brain
- Arthritis
- Stomach ulcers
- Helping skin heal after surgery
- Headaches
- Eye problems
- Gall stones
- Muscle problems
- Asthma

TOXIC EFFECT OF DMSO.

The toxic effect of DMSO is a topic that has led to the scientific study of DMSO, but it might excite you to note that DMSO is of low toxicity compared to many other drugs. The toxic effect of DMSO differs in intensity, dosage, and administration. There are differences in the effects of DMSO and it all depends only on the dosage and method of application. Using DMSO quantity higher than 50% in the blood leads to the development of haemolysis (destruction of red blood cell), while injecting (intravenous) directly with the syringe can cause irritation and cramps.

The LD50 values found in monkeys showed that 880 grams of skin or 320 grams of intravenous fluid could lead to 50% of deaths in people.

The most common complaints related with the use of DMSO are;

- Respiratory odors such as;

- Garlic-like taste,
- Erythema,
- Thirst,
- Occasional pruritus associated with cutting therapy,
- And diarrhea.

In the human body;

- Headaches,

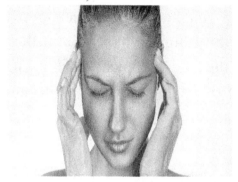

- Nausea,
- Dizziness,
- And drowsiness is stated and it is also assumed that animals may have similar experience.

Urea modified DMSO help to measure some of these side effects. Urea-modified DMSO comprises 60 parts DMSO, 20 parts urea, and 20 parts water. This formula helps reduce the garlic or sulfur odor in the breath as well as mild irritation, pruritus and thirst experience.

Using intravenous method for administering DMSO, it was found that there was no increased daily recurrence of toxins. Injury to the blood vessels as a result of DMSO usage is clearly relative to the application of DMSO and the number of constant injections.

Application of DMSO in the vein should not **exceed 50%** or the implanted vessel may be severely damaged thereby causing fibrosis, inflammation of the blood vessels, and/or thrombi in the arteries. Prompt administration of DMSO to the vein can cause seizures. Local muscle response to subcutaneous or intramuscular injection is directly related to the intensity and total volume of DMSO used.

Responses reported as it regards these injections include inflammation, bleeding, gelatinous (sticky), and reactions to edematous tissue (a swollen caused by blood in the body tissue). A lot of chemical changes connected to the use of DMSO are related to damages affected by red blood cells.

This particular hemolytic effect is dosage related and is characterized by DMSO injected in a high concentration or large quantity. Pulmonary changes related with the orthodox administration of DMSO are uncommon but with the fatal doses of DMSO used, development of pulmonary edema (swelling) begins to occur.

The emergence of pulmonary edema is related to heart failure and hypertension, narrowing of blood vessels, and blood stasis. The most important aspect of DMSO toxicity involves local tissue reactions. DMSO penetrates through the skin swiftly and results in vasodilation (widening of blood vessel) and erythema (redness of the skin) in comparison to the amount of DMSO used.

Although these changes are not permanent, but occlusive dressing should be avoided when using the DMSO. Conclusively, it is evident that DMSO toxicity is minimal when used in standard medical dosage and quantity. Toxic effects are often seen with very high dosage and concentration tests. Because of the toxic evidence, certain precautionary measures should be taken when using DMSO, including the appropriate and safe doses, concentrations, and directions for DMSO usage and appropriate patient selection.

Patients with history of blood related disease, kidney disease, seizures, pregnancy, skin disorders, liver issues (hepatic) or pulmonary disease should be carefully evaluated, and should ensure that the beneficial effects of DMSO surpasses the potential hazard effects.

CHAPTER SIX.

USING DMSO THERAPHY FOR TREATING AILMENTS.

DMSO can be used across a wide arrangement of conditions. DMSO is often times considered for rapid treatment of basically any ailment. DMSO is actually an essential healer regardless of what the ailment may be. To get the best outcome, one must have an understanding and knowledge of when to use it as well as how to use it.

- **<u>DMSO THERAPY FOR AMYLIODOSIS.</u>**

Amyloidosis is a group of degenerative diseases such as primary (if not concomitant) or secondary AA (if associated with an incurable or recurrent disease) disease which can be contagious such as tuberculosis, leprosy, or inflammatory form such as rheumatoid arthritis. It has a wide range of symptoms depending on where the amyloid deposit is accumulated in the body and it can be similar to many other diseases such that other conditions are often assumed in its stead. It is most times difficult to diagnose, particularly at its early stage of development. It poses several effects on internal organs which may affect one side of the body or one organ. Systemic amyloidosis can adversely affect various unrelated organs in the body which in most cases lead to the death of its victim.

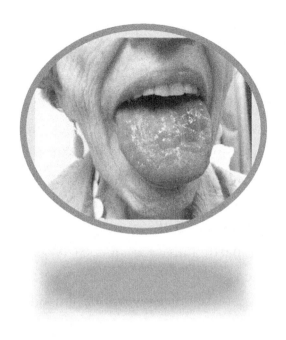

The common treatment for amyloidosis consists mostly of steroids and chemotherapy as well as stem cell transplants but these treatments don't give maximum success. On the other hand, no finding has revealed any contrary reaction to the treatment of amyloidosis using DMSO but a significant improvement has been reported.

For the management of amyloidosis and other related symptoms, DMSO can be taken either orally, applied topically or intravenously alongside other treatments for more effective outcome.

From research, it was discovered that regular oral intake of DMSO treatment of about 7grams to 15grams a day given to 3 patients having amyloidosis case of Familial Mediterranean Fever (FMF), 3 patients with a case of idiopathic amyloidosis (amyloidosis without an underlying cause) and 7 patients having a case of secondary amyloidosis lingering for about 7 to16 months, produced no relevant effect on the first two cases.

However, a fantastic improvement of the renal function was recorded in the 7 patients with a secondary amyloidosis following 3-6 months of administering DMSO therapy. This has been shown to have a 30% to 100% increase in creatinine (a waste product produced by muscles from the breakdown of a compound called creatine) clearance and a decrease in proteinuria (increased levels of protein in the urine).

Regular application of DMSO helped to maintain this balance with no severe side effects except mild nausea and unpleasant respiratory odor which was a major concern for patients. Haven done this research, a conclusion was drawn; that administering DMSO orally, extensively increases life expectancy and this was justified by all patients with cases of secondary amyloidosis.

Dosage Application;
Topically apply *50% to 100%* DMSO concentration once a day for a period of 3 months.

- **DMSO THERAPY FOR TREATING ARTHRITIS.**

Arthritis is an inflammation of one or more joints in the body which may cause pain or stiffness in most cases. Arthritis most times can be mild with minor pain and some of it can be severe. Arthritis is one of the major causes of disability and loss of mobility for people above age 65.

Regular treatment for arthritis is usually a combination of painkillers to help reduce the pains associated with it. The patient might feel relieved of the pain at some point but it may also worsen the situation at the same time.

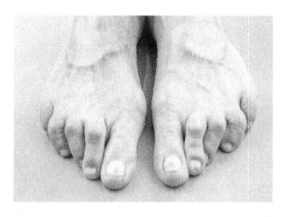

Nevertheless, patients with treated cases of arthritis as well as the doctors who treated those patients generally succumbed to the fact that DMSO is the most potent therapeutical treatment for arthritis noting that there's always an immediate relief after using DMSO.

First, DMSO reduces the pain and muscle aches felt around the joints, and blood circulation also increases which helps to transport the needed nutrients to the affected area. It provides natural sulfur to the damaged joints and also decreases swelling or inflammation.

Irrespective of the underlying cause of the joint pain; whether osteoarthritis (breakdown of one or more joints), rheumatoid arthritis (inflammation or swelling of the joints), juvenile rheumatoid arthritis (arthritis in children), or lupus arthritis (arthritis in small joints), DMSO can help relieve you of this condition.

It helps promote joint mobility as well as reducing inflammation and pain. It additionally helps in the management of amyloidosis; an exorbitant development of protein in organs related to rheumatoid arthritis.

It is ideal to orally take 1 teaspoon of DMSO in 5ounces of refined water or juice. Take once every day for the curation of joint pain. It is likewise a smart thought to utilize the DMSO and vitamin C combination for a quick and more increased relief of inflamed tissues.

Dosage Application;

For treating osteoarthritis: ***25% DMSO*** gel/liquid can be applied 3 times daily and ***45.5%*** DMSO solution can be applied topically 4 times daily for about 21 days.

You can also take ***1 teaspoon*** of DMSO with about 5 ounces of treated water or juice once a day to relief joint pains. You can as well use DMSO alongside ***vitamin C*** for quick relief of inflammation.

- **<u>DMSO THERAPY FOR TREATING ACHES AND NERVE PAIN.</u>**

DMSO produces a form of relief from several forms of pains ranging from muscle pains, pains from injury, nerve pains, tooth aches and also pains from inflammations.

However, there's bound to be fluctuation in the outcome considering different individual's body uniqueness. DMSO is best effective when combined with other medications as it regards treating pains; for example, using DMSO alongside CBD oil (cannabidiol) to relief muscle pain and nausea feelings or using

DMSO topically with herbal wolfsbane (Arnica montana) to reduce muscle pain. Store about 16 ounces of 99.9% of pure DMSO water.

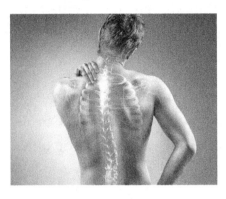

This works best in cases where the DMSO concentration level is between *70% - 90%* thereby having a combination of 70% DMSO and 30% undiluted water, or 90% DMSO concentration and 10% undiluted water. Haven gotten this combination, you can apply the substance directly on the skin using your fingers.

Although experts recommended photographing DMSO to the affected area directly but rubbing it on the skin has proven to have a more improving effect with a lasting duration. In all types of pain-related illnesses, victims have consistently reported immediate reduction in pain using topical application of DMSO or otherwise. In some cases, this may be combined with other analgesic medicines to get lasting pain relief.

Dosage Application;

DMSO should be applied widely around the region where the pain for proper relief; in a case of knee pains, it is advisable to apply DMSO *6 inches below*, above and around the knee area topically. Doing this, will help reduce the skin irritation effect and also aid a quick and lasting recovery.

For a first-time user, you can use about 50% solution of DMSO to know its effects on the pain and the body generally after which, you can increase the percentage as much as you deem fit and necessary. How long and frequency of usage to obtain maximum result it solely your decision to make.

To treat nerve pains, 50% of DMSO solution should be used 4 times a daily for about 3 weeks to obtain a maximum result.

- **DMSO FOR SPORT INJURIES.**

Sport injuries are injuries that occur when you engage in sports or exercise. It can be due to excessive training, lack of training, and unsuitable form or methods. Failure to warm up tends to increase the risk of sports injuries.

Avoiding injuries during sports and athletic situations is almost impossible considering various activities involved ranging from track and field events, fights, football, basketball, weight lifting and a host of others and these injuries may range from mild to severe.

However, every effort can be made towards minimizing the effects of these injuries and also enhance the speedy recovery as fully as possible. DMSO happens to be one effective treatment for these injuries and its best used for sports-related conditions such as, severe bruising, cuts, broken bones as well as tennis elbow dislocation. Having knowledge of how to use this therapy is of paramount importance as this will help hasten the healing process.

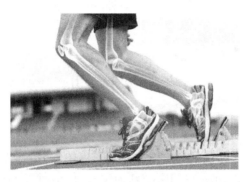

Using a *70%* concentration of DMSO is highly recommended as a potent drug which helps enhance the recovery process and restore muscle strength. Therefore, athletes are advised to add DMSO to their First Aid or Medical aid kits considering its therapeutic benefits.

Dosage Application;

- For severe conditions, apply *70% DMSO* concentration topically for about 2-8 hours immediately after the injury happens.

- Continue to apply it every *4-6 hours* daily for a period of 4 weeks. Although some athletes combine 80% concentration of DMSO with cortisone or 20 percent peppermint oil nevertheless DMSO works alone and athlete can get back to their activities after a while.

- **DMSO FOR BRAIN INJURIES.**

Brain Injury is a disorder of the normal brain function that can be caused by a blow to the head, fall, auto crash, industrial accident, a sudden and violent head striking an object or when an object hits the skull and enters the brain tissue.

Below are some of the clinical signs that make a difference in a normal brain function:

- Loss of consciousness
- Memory loss (amnesia)
- Central nerve deficits such as muscle weakness, blurred vision, changes in speech
- Changes in attitude such as distraction, low thinking or concentration difficulty

The symptoms of brain injury may be mild, moderate, or severe, depending on the severity of the brain damage. Minor cases can lead to small changes in mood or consciousness. Serious cases can lead to long-term coma or even death.

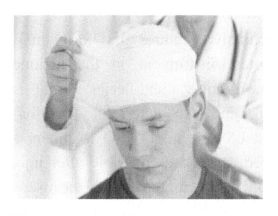

Most times, brain injuries may be difficult to treat using conventional medicine methods. Although, Barbiturates and mannitol are considered the best obtainable treatment for such brain injuries, but researches have shown that DMSO is a better therapy option that supersedes other forms of treatment.

This conclusion was made when a group of patients with brain injuries received barbiturates and mannitol treatment and their brain pressure remained elevated.

However, when 40% concentration of DMSO was administered to these same patients within 3 minutes to 5 minutes, the pressure reduced to normal.

The distinctive features of DMSO make it a very potent instrument in the treatment of severe head injuries and because brain tissue is so weak and can deteriorate rapidly when deprived of oxygen, DMSO treatment should be started as soon as possible after injury. At such, DMSO treatment should be used as an emergency medication by medical personnel which should be applied to the injured head when the patient arrives the hospital. If there are long delays in treatment it usually results to permanent damage to the brain function.

Severe head injuries are usually treated with a simple drip of up to **5gram per kg** of the patient's body weight and this is monitored for about 24 hours to check for any toxic side effects. After the first 24 hours, the dosage can be reduced to **2g to 3g per kg** of the body weight daily.

Another cause of death or disability from head injuries is when blood gathers and begins to compress the brain or when water gathers in the brain and puts pressure on important areas of the brain.

The DMSO treatment used will help improve blood flow that will aid the vascular system evacuate excess blood from the cranial cavity and remove excess fluid. Children with brain injuries can also be treated orally with *50% concentration of DMSO.*

- **DMSO THERAPY FOR TREATING BURNS.**

Burn is an injury to the skin or tissue damage caused by heat, sunburn, radioactivity, electrical or chemical contact. Its treatment depends on the area and the extent of the damage. Burns may be minor; such as sunburn or small scald which can be treated in the comfort of the home or it may be severe/life-threatening that may require emergency medical attention.

A comparative study carried out by a therapist far back 1985 with some victims of burn injuries using DMSO treatment against other burn therapeutic agents like Nitrofurazone, Trimecaine and Monomycin, found out that DMSO was higher in terms of its therapeutic effect and also helped decrease, dissolve and hindered the formation and contraction of scar tissues which remained after the burn healed.

DMSO can also build up skin cells, promoting damage to blocked or damaged arteries that are not conducive to oxygen delivery. Excessive blood supply is problematic due to the fact that if the skin tissues are not supplied with oxygen for a long time; most significant injuries and extra time recovery will take.

In providing tissues with the needed oxygen and reducing inflammatory responses, DMSO help speed up the healing process.

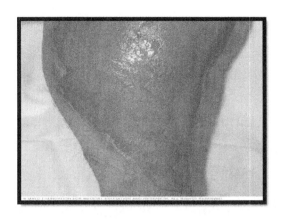

DMSO solution for treating burns is made from a combination of about *50% DMSO* concentration with *50% aloe vera* **gel** which is administered immediately the burn occurs and subsequently for 3 hours. After a while, it can be used in the same way from time to time over the next two days.

Dosage Application;

Topically apply *50% concentration* of DMSO and *50% aloe vera gel* mixture every 3 hours for 3-5 days depending on the degree of the burns.

- **DMSO THERAPY FOR TREATING CANCER.**

Over years, DMSO has been used in the treatment of cancer with maximum positive results. Considering its chemotherapy potentials and its usefulness in several other areas has made one of the most important therapy for treating cancer.

DMSO helps improve blood supply by opening small blood vessels. DMSO as a healing agent on its own is a major anti-cancer therapy talk more of when combined with other anti-cancer drugs. All of these numerous relevant properties combined into a single product indicates that DMSO is a potent therapy for treating cancerous ailments.

From a study on cancer carried out in Chile in which DSMO was combined with amino acid as well as cyclophosphamide and was applied on about *65 cancer patients*, it was recorded that majority if not all the patients on chemotherapy should add DSMO as part of their treatment as a matter of necessity.

The combination of DMSO drugs has a strong anti-splitting function (ability to destroy cancer cells) due to its potential to penetrate DMSO properties. It greatly reduces and sometimes eradicate the toxic effects of Cyclophosphamide, (a chemical agent used mainly in long-term therapy procedures) and at the same time improves the positive effects of chemotherapy.

Dosage Application;
To prevent contrary effects of cancer treatment with medical supervision, topically apply *77% to 90% DMSO* solution every 3-8 hours for 10 to 14 days.

- **DMSO THERAPY FOR DIABETES.**

As a matter of necessity, it is important for DMSO to be included as part of the standard treatment for all diabetic patients because both diabetic neuropaths (a major problem in older adults with cases of diabetes), Type 1 and 2 (usually known as insulin-dependent, or adult onset diabetes) patients has recorded positive results haven used DMSO as part of their treatment regimen.

Diabetes is widely known as a severe ailment with the potential to cause damaged heart and further result in stroke, heart attack and others. From research, it is discovered that diabetic retinopathy (damage to the blood vessels in the tissue at the back of the eye) is the cause of about 2.6% blindness cases recorded across the globe and this is as a result of long-term damage to small blood vessels in the retina and it happens to be the major underlying cause of kidney failure alongside decreased blood circulation.

Also, diabetic neuropathy (nerve damage that affects the feets and legs) is a risk factor for foot numbness, infections to the limb which in most severe cases leads to total amputation.

Prevention should be the ultimate goal in certain cases because a delay treatment might lead to further complications. There's possibility of preventing most diabetic related cases that leads to amputation with regular DMSO treatment.

Dosage Application;

Topically apply DMSO gel/liquid 3 times daily on the affected area;

Drink *1 teaspoon* of DMSO solution every evening after dinner following your diabetic diet plan and exercise for about 6 months depending on the diagnosis.

- **DMSO THERAPY FOR DIGESTIVE PROBLEMS.**

DMSO can to a great extent lessen the adverse effect of digestive related problems when administered together with aloe vera product. Of course, this might not be the final resolution to the ailment until the major cause(s) of the ailment is discovered and removed or reduced to a conceivable level.

Oftentimes, digestive related ailment can be difficult to diagnosed, analyze and treat on a normal ground. Therefore, the need for doctors to be more observant and make enquires about patient's diet plan, the kind of medications they take and other products used by the patient is very necessary because patients oftentimes don't give a 100% information that are relevant in treating such ailment.

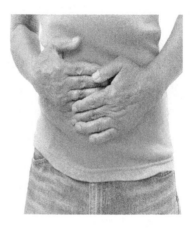

Studies have shown that taking a half teaspoon of DMSO solution alongside 2 ounces of aloe-vera juice in the morning after breakfast and in evening after dinner for 21 days helps reduce gastric related issues and ulcer. DMSO as a therapy has proven potent especially when used on its own, mixed with other antibiotics as well as other infection treatment products.

DMSO has been utilized over the years with outstanding outcomes to move antibiotics to diverse areas in the body system which are oftentimes difficult to reach such as the bone marrow region and the brain.

Digestive related issues of various types can be difficult to treat most timesand significantly more difficult to analyze.

Dosage Application.

Take half a teaspoon of DMSO solution in 1 ounce of an already diluted aloe-vera (you can dilute the aloe vera with 2 ounce of water) twice daily (after breakfast and after dinner). Continue this treatment until you feel relieved of the symptoms.

In the case of symptoms reoccurrence, begin the treatment again for about 2 weeks until all the symptoms dissolves

- **DMSO THERAPY FOR EYE AILMENTS.**

Over the years there has been no evidence that DMSO has not really been proven to have any toxic effect in the eyes over the years. However, research revealed that opthalmologist has recorded great positive outcome haven used DMSO as a therapy in treating and restoring eyes related problems such as glaucoma (decrease pressure within the eyeball), cataract (cloudy natural eye lens), adult vision problems as well as retinal diseases which oftentimes leads to total blindness.

From a research carried out by Dr. Robert Hill of Longview, Washington one of the first set of doctors who used DMSO therapy to treat eye problems which was presented as a report in 1971 at New York Academy of Sciences Conference, revealed that 50% drops of DMSO solution is effective in treating retinitis pigmentosa (when the back wall of the retina is damaged).

This amazing drug (DMSO) can be applied topically for eye problemss such as cataract (cloudy natural clear eye lens) and glaucoma (damage to the eye's optic nerve).

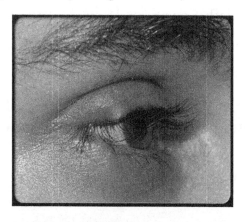

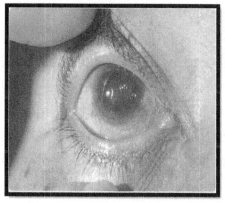

Further studies revealed by doctors showed a significant success recorded by adding a drop of 25mg DMSO solution containing about 2% concentration of saline superoxide dismutase

(SOD) or saline sterile solution using a dropper and apply on both eyes or the affected eye once or twice daily for about 10 days. This will help remove any infection affecting the eyes.

The individual may feel a tingling sensation in the eyes within 30-40 seconds after applying the solution but it will normalize after a while. Using the right proportion and dosage, DMSO has proven to be an effective healing agent in treating eye related problems.

Dosage Application.

Prepare 50% solution of DMSO and drop the liquid in the affected eyes with the aid of an eye dropper and an eye cup (a small oval cup/container which has a cover that is bent to align with the orbit section of the eye that is used in the application of liquid solutions to the eyes), do this for once in a day. You can either use the DSMO solution alone or with vitamin C and glutathion.

Note... *Do not apply DMSO directly to the eyes....... use an eye-drop during application.*

- **DMSO THERAPY FOR TREATING EAR AND HEARING PROBLEMS.**

A lot of children with ear infections are often treated with painful procedures such as piercing the eardrum to release pulse, but combining DMSO solution with other anethestic medicines most times makes the piercing less painful.

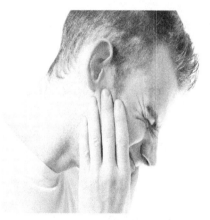

DMSO as a healing agent, is very helpful for any ear related problems, ranging from ear disease, formation of blood clots in the ear causing pain, deafness etc.

Also, patient with middle or inner ear infections can be treated using a combination of both

DMSO solution and antibiotics without piercing the eardrum. From a research carried out in Los Angeles using a family of 6 children who suffered ear infection from infancy, it was discovered that these young children were treated DMSO solution (2 drops of 50% concentration of DMSO).

Also, about 90% of DMSO solution was rubbed around the neck and head region near the affected ear and this gave a great relief.

The mothers of the children, and we need to continue the treatment at home due to the formation of DMSO drops in the ear twice a day, and how to apply it in case of the slightest sign of fear.

And it was simple and effective, with good medical care.

Dosage Application.

Prepare 20% of DMSO solution with either saline solution or pure (undiluted) water. Put the mixture inside an empty eye drop container and apply 1-2 drops in the affected ear once a day.

If there's any pain in the ear after applying this solution, you have stop using it for at least a day to enable the ear respond adequately to the treatment.

However, if the pain continues, you should stop using DMSO treatment and an ear expert (doctor) for proper examination and further treatments.

- **DMSO THERAPY FOR FUNGUS INFECTIONS.**

Over the years, DMSO has been considered an effective healing agent considering its healing potentials embedded in it. It is an important healing agent in treating fungus infection when used either alone or combined with other antibiotics such as griseofulvin to treat ringworms, toenail infection (mycotic), athlete's foot, etc.

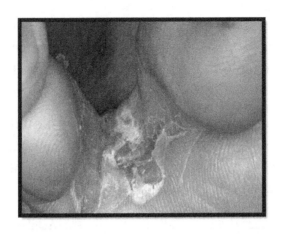

Dosage Application.

Combine DMSo with iodine to make 90% concentrated solution and apply topically on the affected area every 4 hours for 3 days. You can also seek medical guidance when using this solution.

- **DMSO THERAPY FOR HAIR GROWTH AND SCALP PROBLEMS.**

For several years now DMSO has proven to be a good product for enhancing hair growth and treating hair related issues as well as recovering hair lost as a result of chemotherapy (for cancer patients).

The main reason for using DMSO to enhance hair growth is because it is an outstanding therapy which helps widen the small blood vessels in the scalp and further enhance blood flow as well as other important nutrients to the hair follicles.

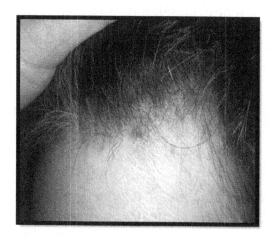

This therapy was applied by an 80-year-old man in Oklahoma who has sticky substance spilling from his head. After much diagnosis and examination by a specialist, it was discovered that he has an infection under the head skin and a possible remedal option was made available; which is to remove the affected head skin.

However, he rejected the offer because the option seems extreme for the old patient and DMSO ointment was further recommended. After applying this ointment for about 6 months, it was recorded that the affected area healed up. From this illustration, one could imagine the healing potency embedded in DMSO.

All you need is just 50% solution of DMSO, apply it on affected hair and scalp but in the case of sensitive skin, it's advisable you use just 40% solution and wash it off with shampoos and conditioners. Some persons use this once a week while others use it everyday depending on your skin sensitivity. DMSO helps enhance hair radiance and thickness, it makes the hair grow longer and improves its development.

Note... *Ensure you remove any external products such as spray, mousse, gel etc from the hair before applying the solution.*

Dosage Application;
Apply 50% concentration DMSO solution topically on the scalp 2 times daily for 3 months.

- **DMSO THERAPY HEADACHES AND MIGRAINES.**

Headaches as an ailment differs in type and virtually everyone experience at some point in our lives. Oftentimes, it occurs as a result of muscle contraction in the neck, changes in the blood veins entering the head and the way our body responds to stressful situations.

Aside regular treatment people use for headaches, DMSO has also been very useful in treating headaches with great positive outcome over the years without any negative effect.

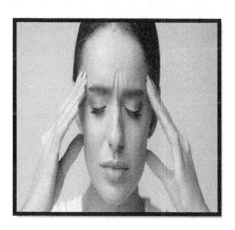

However, it's been observed that when migraine headaches are treated in an advanced stage, they do not respond promptly to treatment but if they are treated within the early stage, the condition is often reversed with DMSO as shown in many patients.

DMSO is usually applied within 24 hours of pain in the upper back, neck, or both. Although, this therapy can be more effective when applied intravenously either through injection or the patient add it to juice or water and drink at least 4 times daily for 21 days. All you need to do is pour small quantity of water into a cup and add equal quantity of DMSO solution to the water (50% water and 50% DMSO) and then drink.

For stronger solution considering the severity of the pain, you can mix ***25% water and 75% DMSO.***

Note... *when mixing, ensure you pour water in the cup first before adding DMSO.*

In most cases, DMSO help prevent the onset of migraine at such it is necessary to administer

DMSO immediately you notice any slight pain in the head.

Dosage Application;

Apply a mixture of **50% water and 50% DMSO**; you can add aloe vera gel to it. Measure 1 teaspoon of the mixture and run it between the two eyes near your forehead, on the neck, and the throat area.

Do this every 1 hour for 3 hours. You can stop using it once you notice any relief before the stated 3 hours if not, continue using it 3 times daily until the pain diminish.

- **DMSO THERAPY FOR INFLAMMATION.**

Inflammation on the other hand, the body's response to injury or destruction of tissue damaged by disease or injury. It is strongly associated with symptoms of pain, swelling, fever, redness, and loss of function.

DMSO as mentioned earlier is a potent anti-inflammatory drug used to relieve inflammation and it is recommendable for other inflammatory problems. It can reduce all symptoms of inflammation like swelling, normalize temperature, and reduction in pain as reported by patients.

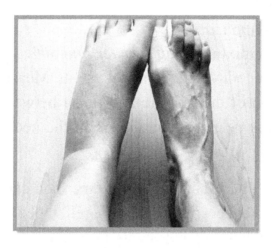

Also, DMSO help increase the activity of cortisol (the body's stress hormone) produced in the adrenal glands (small structures attached to the top of each kidney) as a natural anti-inflammatory hormone. Steroid drug like cortisone that's oftentimes used in place of the natural cortisol produced by the body has been of greet benefit to patients when used for a short period of time but can be life threatening when used for a longer duration.

However, DMSO has proven to be not only effective as an anti-inflammatory agent in itself but with no side effects as opposed other steroid and non-steroid anti-inflammatory medicine. From a study conducted at an orthopedic clinic in California, it was discovered that many arthritic patients who were previously treated with cortisone, NSAIDS, or both were treated again DMSO alongside diet and exercise.

Dosage Application;

Apply **40%** concentration of DMSO topically 3 times daily for 10-12 days. You can increase the dosage depending on how delicate the affected area is.

- **DMSO THERAPY FOR MENTAL ILLNESS AND RETARDATION.**

DMSO is a very powerful and widely used drug in the treatment of mental retardation and down syndrome. In cases where the patient's intelligent quotient (IQ) is less than 50, the facial features of the body differ from normal and the psychological symptoms are affected.

Sometimes DMSO is administered alone but in most cases, it is combined with amino acids, vitamins, or other products. DMSO management practices vary; that is, it's mode of application differs. It can be given orally; the patient can mix it in water, juice or milk, injected directly into the skin or apply it topically (rub) on the skin.

DMSO is a very potent drug for treating with serious psychiatric disorders including schizophrenia, late psychoses, obsessive-compulsive neurosis, anxiety disorders, and other psychological issues for several decades and the resulting effects has been amazing.

Note.... *Before using DMSO as a treatment, previous medications should be stopped for at least a week.*

Dosage Application;
<u>Intravenously:</u> Apply 5ml muscle injections of **50% -80% DMSO** concentration concentration. This should be done 2 to 3 times per day but in more severe cases, 5 injections daily can be administered.

People who present with minor symptoms can be given few drops of 50% DMSO concentration.

- **DMSO THERAPY FOR SKIN AILMENT.**

Skin illnesses such as skin ulcers can occur for a variety of reasons; maybe due to diabetic sores, infected wounds or burns.

The most effective treatment used to achieve good results is DMSO combined with antibiotics and other anti-inflammatory agents as attested to by victims of skin ailment.

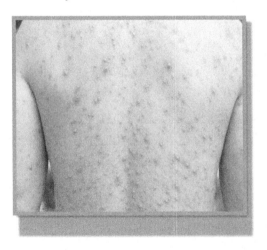

DMSO is helpful in combating aging effect, treating scars, reducing wrinkles, and other skin problems including acne. In a bid to get a standard facial look one must be cautious when combining DMSO with other skin care products as this will help protect the skin from toxins.

To obtain an optimum result, it's ideal to use DMSO solution of 40% concentration mixed with pure water or aloe vera gel.

Dosage Application;

To apply the lotion on your skin, mix DMSO, aloe-vera gel and eucalyptus oil together and rub it on the affected area 2 times daily for 5days.

- **DMSO THERAPY FOR SHINGLES AND HERPES.**

Shingles is a viral infection that causes a painful rash. Although shingles can occur anywhere in the body, it usually appears as a single line of blisters that wraps around the left or right side of the victim's body.

Although it's not a life-threatening condition, but can be very painful. Medicinal vaccines can aid the reduction of its associated risks and immediate remedial actions which can help diminish the shingles effect as well as its complications possibility.

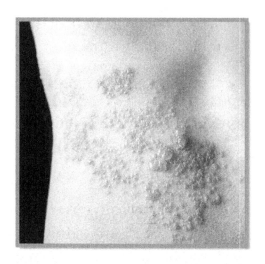

Herpes Sister (shingles) comes from the same virus that causes chickenpox. Most of the time it lasts for few weeks. It's symptoms rangws from; pain, burning sensation, numbness or tingling, sensitivity to touch, red rash that begins a few days after the pain, fluiid-filled blisters that break open and crust over, Itching and several others.

Although there's a vaccine for treating shingles but it doesn't give a permanent cure, as there's every tendency of the ailment resurfacing after some time.

However, DMSO often creates an interesting effect when used for the treatment of cold sores a similar effect of shingles virus.

Dosage Application;

Get a mixture of 30% DMSO solution and *10 to 15ppm (parts per million)* of colloidal silver in a bottle; you can use undiluted water as well.

Constantly apply it topically on the affected area few times daily in a lower dosage. You can increase the dosage with time depending on your skin sensitivity with the solution.

You can also apply a mixture of *5% to 40%* of idoxuridine and DMSO solution topically 2 days after the rash appears every 4 hours for about 4 days.

- **DMSO FOR STROKE, SPINAL CORD INJURIES.**

DMSO has been known over the years as a superior treatment for stroke. When used appropriately, it can save the lives of many stroke victims by providing immediate medical attention.

Delay in application can lead to very serious consequences which in most cases might be irreversible and further result in chronic brain injury/damage or death.

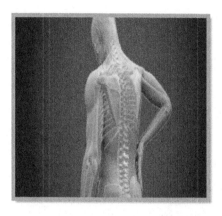

Prompt use of DMSO in the event of a minor stroke may help reduce the possibility of any permanent damage but in the case of a severe stroke, it helps prevent chronic/permanent disability or death in victims.

Considering the numerous healing benefits of DMSO, it should be used to treat all patients with a stroke because it has the ability to cross the blood-brain barrier, which acts as a protective barrier between blood and brain circulation.

DMSO helps other blood vessels to take up the function of any damaged blood vessels, thus saving the life of a stroke victim as well as effective in treating spinal ulcers without any harmful side reaction.

When DMSO is injected into the body or skin, using an IV or oral method. It flows into the body, cross the brain barrier, melts the stroke causal agent (clot), restore blood circulation and thus prevents paralysis in victims.

Although IV is well recommended, because there is a high rate of blood flow in the traumatized region.

Dosage Application;

Treatment should begin immediately the incident occurs. Patients should topically apply DMSO solution twice daily

- **Intravenously:** Inject DMSO solution once a day
- **Orally:** Take 1 teaspoonful of DMSO solution in juice twice daily for 2 weeks.

CHAPTER SEVEN.

POSSIBLE SIDE EFFECTS OF DMSO.

The side effects of DMSO differs depending on individual body system. It ranges from redness that usually occurs when the solution applied which disappears after several application.

Among 25-30% of people who use DMSO solution, a burning sensation is felt on spot where the solution is applied while some experience allergic reactions as well as headaches. Few patients report;

- Slight itching
- blistering,
- Skin inflammation; dry, red or swollen skin.
- Foul odor in the body or mouth, nausea feeling etc.

When DMSO is use orally, there's tendency for the individual to experience;

- Woozy feeling
- Drowsiness,

- Nausea/vomiting
- Diarrhea,
- Constipation.

Note... *that all of the above mentioned are just side effects with no toxic reactions.*

However, patients with Asthma, liver or kidney ailment, diabetes. For precaution should not administer DMSO solution without first consulting the doctor.

DMSO MIXTURE QUANTITY & DOSAGE.

- **For 50/50 percent solution:** Get 1 or 2 teaspoons of distilled water, aloe-vera juice or colloidal silver with 1 or 2 teaspoons of 99% DMSO and mix them together in a container the apply the mixture on the affected area daily.

- **70/30 percent solution:** Mix 70% undiluted water, aloe-vera juice or colloidal silver with 30% DMSO together and use this once or twice a day.

- **10/90 percent solution:** Mix 10% portion of DMSO with 90% distilled water, aloe-vera juice or colloidal silver to get an ointment or cream solution.

CHAPTER EIGHT.

PRECAUTIONARY MEASURES OF DMSO FOR PREGNANT WOMEN AND NURSING MOTHERS.

DMSO medication, like all unofficial drugs, should be avoided both as a breastfeeding mother or expectant mother because it is better to be on a safer side and take precautions while taking other prescribed medicines for the benefit of the child as direct use of DMSO can pose a negative effect on the unborn child or the newborn through breastfeeding.

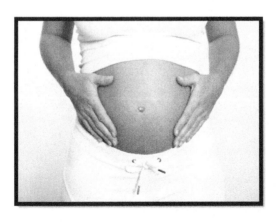

Therefore, pregnant women and breastfeeding mothers should not take DMSO, because less reliable/concrete information is known for its potential effects on the fetus or infant.

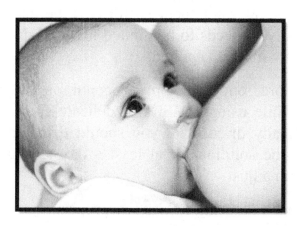

- **REASONS FOR STORING AND MIXING DMSO.**

The great advantage of DMSO can be attributed to the fact that it is a well-formed bipolar molecule, which means that one end of the molecule loves water and the other limit loves fat, making it a global solution.

When applying it on an open wounds or very sensitive areas, it is best to apply a weak solution. You can decide to buy an already mixed solution or you do the mixing yourself with pure water (undiluted water), aloe vera gel/juice or colloidal silver.

One of the major reasons why DMSO is been diluted with other solvent is because it has a dehydrating component so for it to be applied regularly, it needs to be diluted to avoid drying up the skin when applied.

Therefore, one can apply coconut oil on the skin while using DMSO for delicate skin. For an already dried skin, you should discontinue using the solution for at least a day to enable the skin adjust.

Storing and using DMSO appropriately is of paramount importance especially when purchasing an already mixed product; make sure it is stored in the glass container not plastic because the plastic container can emit some chemicals into the DMSO solution thereby transferring harmful toxins into the bloodstream system which may lead to other ailments.

So, while treating an ailment we must be careful not to bring in other ailments to our body.

OTHER PRECAUTIONARY MEASURES IN THE USE OF DMSO.

Proper use of DMSO will produce positive results results and it'stendency to create risk is very small. Therefore, there is a need to be cautious about its usage as well as other medications. Dimethylsulfoxide (DMSO) may be effective for people with any of the following conditions:

- **Skin Irritation.**

The most common issue with DMSO after usage is redness of the skin, tingling sensation, swelling, peeling of the skin or burn. Although these contrareactions are minor but to reduce the effect, the individual should lower the daily dosage used.

Therefore, regular adjustment of the recommended percentage of solutions to suit your skin type and body will be of great benefit.

Note... *DMSO can also cause reactions to paintings, at such it shouldn't be use on a* *tattooed spot. It can take penetrate the color into the body, which of course may be harmful considering that most tattoo inks have harmful chemicals in their content.*

- **<u>Clean the Skin.</u>**

Before applying DMSO on the skin, ensure the affected area is properly cleaned because anything that DMSO comes into contact with, can be transmitted into the body.

Therefore, it is necessary clean up thoroughly with soap and water, or perhaps, you can bath before using the solution.

In a case of exercising and sweating, ensure to clean the sweat off the skin first, before applying DMSO because the skin absorbs waste products, especially through sweat which oftentimes contains toxic substances that can be harmful when re-introduced.

To be on a safer side, shower before applying DMSO solution.

- **Taste of DMSO.**

DMSO is an amazing particle with so many benefits, however, it is a combination of sulfur compound and the taste of sulfur is not suitable in the mouth but it shouldn't restrain us from using it because it is undoubtedly helpful.

Therefore, in a bid to reduce the harsh flavor, it is recommended that DMSO should be diluted with either pure water, aloe vera juice, orange juice or grape juice as used by some persons.

- **Dangers For Children.**

DMSO can be used on children but on a restricted basis and administering this solution on children in high dosage or for a long duration is not recommendable

In clinical cases, organs and stem cells meant for transplant into children as well as adults are preserved through the use of DMSO. Nevertheless, applying high dosage of DMSO is not suitable for children because they quickly separate the tissues of the nervous system.

- **Dosage Measures.**

Administering DMSO in appropriate dosage is important and this helps with self-education. The rate at which DMSO is used varies, depending on the situation at hand. However, you must understand that combining the right doses for a specific ailment at a consistent rate will bring you the best results.

- **DMSO With Alcohol.**

It is very important not to drink alcohol while using DMSO. Alcohol often known as carcinogen (phase 1) is toxic to the liver, so drinking it is contrary to the purpose of achieving a better health.

When alcohol and DMSO are taken concurrently, DMSO tends to fight the harmful effect of the alcohol rather than taking care of the ailment....as such, DMSO act as a defensive agent to the alcohol effect leaving the ailment untreated.

- **DMSO And It's Odour.**

Pure DMSO is odorless, but when mixed with various substances, sulfur-like odor can be detected.

At the initial stage of DMSO which is DMS (dimethyl sulfide) through decomposition, it emits a sulfur-like odor with a garlic or onions smell. Although few persons may not have this smell after using DMSO while others may have it.

Using DMSO to treat mouth and gum infections can cause bad breath. Due to this bad smell, treatment can be done at night so that by the next morning the odor would have reduced.

CHAPTER NINE.

CONCLUSION.

In all of the above, it is very important to watch your body system when using a product like DMSO to make sure you are using it properly and staying safe.

Normally, the benefits associated with using DMSO will be felt in the first 21 days but may take longer time in chronic/acute cases. So, the patients are more likely to continually apply it for at least six weeks or more before the onset of a noticeable effect, with many patients still reporting significant relief that they have never experienced in any other treatment.

However, some patients with chronic conditions experience immediate pain relief, which may take six to eight weeks, and in few cases 6 months for complete change depending on the level of the pain and the patient involved. It is very important that DMSO as a therapy is used under the guidance of a medical professional.

DMSO benefits human body cells, tissues, and organs in a diverse positive avenue, a 21st-century healing agent that demonstrates various approach to the disease treatment with great importance. It is not just as a drug for a particular ailment, but as a remedy that normalizes body system function as a whole.

DMSO has proven to be perhaps a major product for reducing human suffering. It is beneficial in treating various kind diseases when used alone or combined with other products and has been shown to be part of the safest drug. Aside the fact that some persons tend to abuse it at the early stage, no death nor toxic reactions has been recorded from its usage.

It's necessary for medical practitioners to know more about DMSO thereby incorporating it's use into other medical practice. In some cases, the specialist may not know what is happening to the patient as symptoms presented and test results may be unclear.

However, it is well-known that something is undoubtedly my right. At such, DMSO may be helpful without any negative resultant effect.

DMSO is seen as an innumerable clinical or medical useful agent because of continuous clinical evolvement but it's development is being hindered because some medical specialists don't imbibe the fact that a particular drug or medicine can heal or bring relief to various types of disease and ailment.

Yes, familiarizing ourselves with DMSO is good but we must not undermine the precautionary measures needed to be taken, as this will help ensure we get the maximum result we desire. Different diseases come with different methods of treatments. Therefore, medicine concentration, dosage and procedures for application should be known by those using it.

THE END.

Made in the USA
Monee, IL
24 September 2022